T0147598

ABS-olutely Simple

Brian Bebley

iUniverse, Inc.
New York   Bloomington

ABS-olutely Simple

Copyright © 2010 by Brian Bebley

All rights reserved. No part of this book may be used or reproduced by any means, graphic, electronic, or mechanical, including photocopying, recording, taping or by any information storage retrieval system without the written permission of the publisher except in the case of brief quotations embodied in critical articles and reviews.

You should not undertake any diet/exercise regimen recommended in this book before consulting your personal physician. Neither the author nor the publisher shall be responsible or liable for any loss or damage allegedly arising as a consequence of your use or application of any information or suggestions contained in this book.

iUniverse books may be ordered through booksellers or by contacting:

iUniverse
1663 Liberty Drive
Bloomington, IN 47403
www.iuniverse.com
1-800-Authors (1-800-288-4677)

Because of the dynamic nature of the Internet, any Web addresses or links contained in this book may have changed since publication and may no longer be valid. The views expressed in this work are solely those of the author and do not necessarily reflect the views of the publisher, and the publisher hereby disclaims any responsibility for them.

ISBN: 978-1-4502-5091-7 (sc)
ISBN: 978-1-4502-5092-4 (ebk)

Library of Congress Control Number: 2010911824

Printed in the United States of America

iUniverse rev. date: 8/27/2010

I dedicate this to my lovely wife,
Mrs. Sandra Bebley

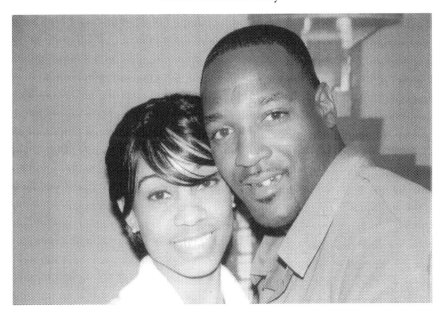

Contents

Introduction

Are you tired of all those fitness books that guarantee you results if you just follow their plan?

I'm assuming you are, because what you are now reading is the truth, and we both share a common goal. Your goal is to get in shape, get ripped, get shredded, and lose weight. My goal is to make sure you get to where you want to be as quickly as possible from the comforts of your own home.

Do you hate to read those self-proclaimed miracle fitness books and get lost in the amount of medical and scientific words and terms they use that supposedly help you with your quest to lose weight?

If you're like me you like to get straight to the point without feeling like you're reading another language. Well, don't worry—this is not one of those books, even though I'm certified in advanced endurance training and in personal training. I'm not here to make myself look overly intelligent. I'm here to cut out all the unnecessary things and get to the meat of the subject. My easy-to-use book is broken down into four parts to help you lose weight and get that washboard stomach you've always wanted. Don't get me wrong—exercising, or putting in work as I like to call it, is a major part of working out, but it's not the most important part of getting the body you desire.

I know that it might come as a surprise to you, but I'm here to inform you that along with the willpower to get in shape, a sound and healthy diet is the most important part of losing weight and staying healthy. Losing weight will enhance your overall appearance, which in term will boost your confidence.

Losing weight will also increase your sex drive. Did you know that a healthy breakfast at the start of your day consisting of eggs and oats, both of which have vitamins like B6 and B12, keeps you going even longer in the sheets and reduces stress? Breakfast is a key component in starting your day and also finishing up the night with memorable moments with your significant other. Even if you don't have time for eggs and oatmeal, there are plenty of choices for healthy cereals that are loaded with vitamins that will help you in that department, but we'll get more into the better sex thing later.

Once you lose the weight you desire you'll feel better and look better. The truth of the matter is that people respond better to healthier-looking people in a work environment as well as in a social setting. Lose weight, get ripped, get in shape, look better, live longer, and feel better—these are some of the benefits of getting in shape. There are also many more, and I'm here to assist you with this process. So stay focused and be consistent.

I'm confident that you will achieve your goal and see the progress you want, so without further ado I wish you good fortune on your journey!

Unlike many of those who write these workout books, I am actually a product of my own system, which is proven to work. These four basic chapters along with hard work will get you the same results that I achieved! Time and *patience* is the key to a successful outcome!

I would also like to add that I'm supplement free, because I would rather go natural and see the long-term results of all my hard work pay off rather than add a bunch of supplements to my diet for immediate results and have a whole series of long-term side effects. This is just my point of view; the choice is always yours. In my personal opinion, nothing good comes fast, but the good things come with time.

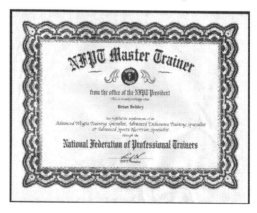

Chapter 1
Dieting and Weight Loss

I agree with many certified dietary nutritionists: Most diets don't work. The correct way to lose weight is to develop a solid eating plan and stick with it.

Diets make you feel tired. They make you hungry, and they don't last long. The reason is that most short-term fad diets cut carbs, protein, or other essential aspects of a sound natural diet to the point where your body sacrifices muscle in the process of losing weight by cannibalization or because you are just not getting the fuel you need for your workout requirements.

Most people lose weight rather quickly when they start these trend diets, which can open up a whole new can of worms when it comes to your health. But ask yourself at what expense you are losing the weight; the truth of the matter is that the weight never stays off, because most of these diets are not intended as a new way of life.

To sum it all up, there's no substitute for healthy eating. Taking in whole foods is something that will benefit you for the rest of your life!

1. Stay away from liquid calories. The calories in sodas, fruit juices, and beer add up quickly. So switch your soda with water. Use low-fat dressing instead of your regular dressing, and cut out artificial sweeteners altogether. Making these small changes can help you reduce your weight in a big way.

2. Stop eating all those processed meats we all love so much. Processing foods takes out all the good stuff like fiber, vitamins, and minerals and replaces them with fats and sugars; you should be getting all your carbs in the form of whole grains, veggies, beans, nuts, and fruits.

3. Consuming your meals in smaller amounts more frequently is a sure way to get your metabolism going at full speed. The reason is that if you break the four to five meals you currently eat into six or seven smaller meals you won't feel as hungry as you usually do between meals, which won't cause you to reach for something bad like a bag of chips. This instead allows your muscles to have and store the fuel they need for your exercise routines. You also burn calories every single time you eat, so doesn't that make more sense than eating those large meals and feeling bloated throughout the day while your body fights to digest those Super Bowl–size meals?

With your new exercise routines you'll need to boost your protein consumption as well; you should be doing this by eating your proteins throughout the day. This will help your body absorb proteins in a more efficient way so you can call on these resources for energy when needed. Carb and protein combinations are the best way to eat; for example, turkey on wheat or tuna salad. Last but not least don't shy away from carbs. I know that might sound a little odd to you, considering the fact that most trend diets tell you to reduce or cut carbs out altogether. But the truth of the matter is that carbs provide the bulk of the energy needed for your workouts. Your body puts out less insulin after about 6:00 PM, so in turn it's harder for your body to break down those carbs at that point. Potatoes, rice, oatmeal, breads, and all other types of starchy complex carbs should be nowhere near your mouth at this time. When you do eat carbs after 6:00 PM they should consist mostly of veggies, things your body can break down more efficiently, such as cucumbers, spinach, lettuce, and broccoli, for example. Those types of veggies are less filling and good for you too.

Did you know that eating more slowly can assist in your weight loss? The faster you eat, the more calories you consume before your brain even gets the memo. The point is that if you're scarfing down pizza by the slice, before you know it you've taken in more calories than are needed for an entire day in one meal. Eating more slowly gives your body time to register that it's consuming food. So your fullness switch kicks on and doesn't allow you to eat as much as when you're scarfing your food down. Eat more slowly; it's not a race!

Sex facts

Remember, I told you I'd get back to the better sex thing! Well, I hope you didn't think I had a secret solution to all your problems. I don't, but you do; let me explain. When it comes to the bedroom, confidence plays a significant part in your performance. If you don't feel good about the way you look you won't put on the performance demanded.

The bottom line is that the better you look, the better you feel about yourself, and when you feel good about yourself, so does everyone around you, including your significant other.

Being overweight can get in the way of your becoming the person you desire to be in the bedroom, because the years of eating incorrectly and not exercising can affect erections or ED, erectile dysfunction. This is caused by clogged arteries that make it almost impossible for the blood you need to flow toward the penis.

The only solution to better sex is a better and healthier lifestyle that consists of eating better and getting enough exercise.

Eating small meals and its benefits

The more you eat in the form of smaller meals the more your body is forced to work and burn calories.

When you eat large meals in an infrequent way throughout the day, especially while sedentary for several hours of each day, your body is doing nothing significant. Your metabolism slows down because not enough frequent meals are being ingested. The body is being starved in the long term.

Now when you start to take in more calories the body jumps into survival mode and thinks it is starving and will store all of these calories as fat and not use them for the body to process.

If you eat small meals throughout the day, the body knows that it's not being starved, so it releases its fat around the clock for bodily functions while at the same time working to digest food that will help to speed up your metabolism.

The glycemic index

The glycemic index shows you how carbs are categorized according to how quickly the body converts them to glucose and pushes them into your blood stream.

The higher a food is on the (GI) chart the faster it's broken down into glucose. Also note that protein, fiber, and fats slow digestion down, so keep that in mind also.

To play it safe eat foods that fall on the low end of the (GI) chart. You can find easy-to-use glycemic indexes just about anywhere on the Internet.

Remember that a dietitian is the only person who can give you an accurate diet plan to suit your workout needs.

High Glycemic
BEVERAGES

Carbonated soft drinks   68
Gatorade   91

BREAD AND GRAIN
PRODUCTS
Oatmeal   61
Grape Nuts cereal   67
Bread, whole wheat   69
Bread, white   70
Cream of wheat   70
Bagels   72
Bran flakes   74
Graham crackers   74
Puffed wheat   74
Cheerios   75
Breakfast bars   76
Total cereal   77
Corn flakes   84

FRUITS
Raisins   64
Watermelon   72
Honey   73

VEGETABLES
Potatoes, microwaved   82
Potatoes, baked   85

Moderate Glycemic
BREAD AND GRAIN
PRODUCTS
Pasta   41
Pumpernickel bread   41
All Bran cereal   42
Muesli, toasted   43
Bulgur   47
Buckwheat (kasha)   54
Popcorn   55
Rice, brown   55
Special K   55
Rice, white   56
Mini-wheats   58
Bran muffins   60

FRUITS
Apple juice, unsweetened   41
Oranges   43
Bananas, overripe   52
Orange juice   57

LEGUMES
Lentil soup   44
Baked beans   48

VEGETABLES
Peas   48
Sweet potatoes   54
Corn   55

Low Glycemic
BREAD AND GRAIN PRODUCTS
Barley   25
Power bar   30–35

DAIRY PRODUCTS
Whole milk   27
Skim milk   32
Yogurt, low-fat, fruit   33
Chocolate milk   34

FRUITS
Cherries   23
Grapefruit   25
Plums   25
Bananas, underripe   30
Peaches   30–40
Apricots, dried   31
Strawberries   32
Apples   36
Pears   36

LEGUMES

Soybeans   18
Kidney beans   27
Lentils   29
Black beans   30
Green beans   30
Soy milk   30
Lima beans   32
Split peas, yellow   32
Chickpeas   32
Pinto beans   39

Dieting facts

Carbohydrates: It is important to note that you will know when you are eating too much soluble fiber when you are experiencing stomach cramps within about twenty to thirty minutes after eating.

Protein: The enzyme pepsin breaks down proteins into smaller proteins (peptides). Once proteins are moved to the small intestine, they're broken down even more by proteases, trypsin, and chymotrypsin into amino acids and absorbable peptides.

(While starting your workout plan you should be consuming at least one gram of protein per pound of body weight to gain muscle mass. Also note that with bumping your protein amount up you need to continue to drink water at each meal to help with digestion.)

Complete proteins need to be ingested every three to four hours to insure the availability of all possible combinations of amino acids for cellular uptake.

Metabolism: A simple way to sum up metabolism is that to lose weight you have to consume fewer calories than you burn. The downside to this is that if you eat too few calories you risk slowing your metabolism down. Eat the right type of calories and you can speed your metabolism up. Eat the wrong types and you run the risk of still gaining weight. So with that in mind you have to start reading the labels of the foods you eat and watching for the recommended serving size. Little do you know that the can of chili you eat for lunch might actually be two servings. This means that you have to double the calorie intake listed on the can to get an accurate calorie intake for the amount you're eating. Start by reducing your portions by half.

For example, if you read the label on the back of a can of your favorite meal you will find the calorie amount, sodium count, sugar, and protein count, but if you look further at the fine print at the top of that label you'll see that the amount listed is usually just for one serving. If that can is two servings, you have to double the amount on the label to see how much you are actually consuming.

Metabolism: Metabolism is the chemical process occurring within living cells or organisms that are necessary for the maintenance of life.

Foods that can set you back

These are just a few items that are detrimental to your diet and weight-loss program. Stay away from foods and drinks that contain these things!

Coffee: Has a negative effect on fluid balance and stimulates nervous activity because of the caffeine it contains.

Chocolate: Has the same effect that coffee does on the body because of its diverted effect and because it has too much sugar.

Salt: Contributes to high blood pressure and contains sodium, causing fluid retention and potassium loss.

Sugar: Absorbed too quickly, causing a rapid rise and fall of blood sugar. Also if eaten too much it can cause fat deposits.

Alcohol: Suppresses nervous function and overworks the liver.

Drugs: All drugs have their effects on the nervous and endocrine systems, which are very delicate and can be seriously impaired.

Tobacco: Nicotine constricts vessels, contributing to high blood pressure; contains carcinogens that destroy respiratory tissues.

Red meat, fried foods, and milk and dairy products: All these products have saturated fats in them because they come from animals; saturated fats contribute to cardiovascular diseases.

Low fiber intake: Leads to poor digestion and poor assimilation of foods and contributes to cancer and metabolic disorders.

Heart rate

220–age (in years) = Max HR

Check pulse for 15 seconds x 4 = Rest HR

Rest HR + [0.60 x (Max HR– Rest HR)] = E x HR

This is the formula you use to get your exercise heart rate (E x HR). Your exercise heart rate should be at least the sum of resting heart rate (Rest HR) plus a percentage of the difference between the age-predicted maximum (Max HR) and resting heart rate (Rest HR).

You must properly measure recovery between sets performed. The higher the recovery rate, the greater the intensity of the workout. Palpate your pulse at the wrist or neck between sets in a seated position. Upon completion of a set while still in the seated position count the numbers of beats in a fifteen-second time period and multiply this number by four to end up with the number of beats per minute. Repeat this process until you are at or below the recommended recovery heart rate. In your case it should be 100–115 bpm or slightly higher. At a heart rate in this area you can achieve general fitness while at the same time building stamina and lean muscle mass.

When it comes to your workout there is a relationship between heart rate and oxygen uptake, which is the best way to measure functional capacity. Therefore as your workout intensity increases, your heart rate increases as well, making it the method of choice for monitoring your workout.

Ten quick tips

1: Eat ninety minutes before you work out.

2: Eat every two to three hours during the day.

3: Eat after you work out; your post-workout window is small, so take advantage of it.

4: Get plenty of rest.

5: Take multi-vitamins/minerals.

6: Drink plenty of water, at least eight to ten cups a day.

7: Ingest fiber; fiber absorbs fat from your digestive tract, and water-insoluble fiber is the best for staying regular.

8: Eat more veggies; the darker green the better.

9: Eat more fish like salmon, mackerel, and tuna.

10: Stay away from fried foods!

Chapter 2
Stretching

Flexibility is the most important part of your training. Far too often people overlook stretching as a part of working out, but in fact it's a very important aspect of working out. Stretching prevents injuries and helps with flexibility. The more flexible you are, the better range of motion you'll have, which will allow for better repetitions and in turn give you a better workout.

When they're healthy, muscles can elongate up to 1.6 times their length, but they generally don't react well with too much stretching. If you hold in a stretch position for too long your muscle instantly protects itself by recoiling. This protects the muscle from ripping. This effect usually kicks in after staying in a stretched position for longer than three minutes.

A stretch should be held for no longer than ten to thirty seconds to provide adequate flexibility and to prepare you for your workout routine.

Take your time with each movement; stretching should be followed by a light warm-up session. I prefer two to three sets of jumping jacks.

Stretch 1

Up, back, and over
This is a three-count routine.

Start in the standing position, arms at your sides. Count one: bring both arms forward and upward. Count two: bring both arms down and back. Count three: bring both arms forward, up, back, and around to complete a full circle.

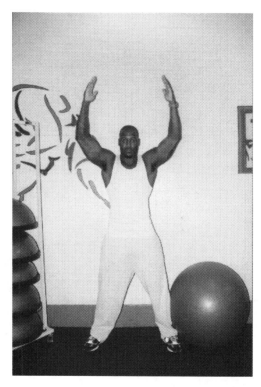

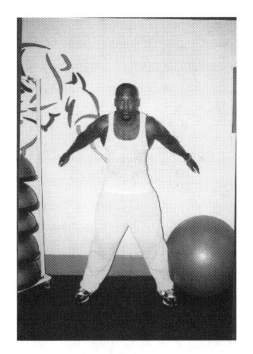

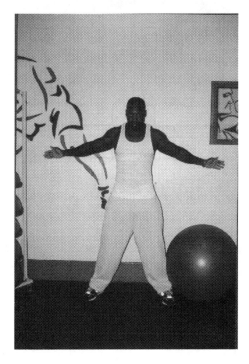

Targets: Shoulders, chest, and back

Stretch 2

Core twist

Start in the seated position, with your hands behind your head. Rotate (twist) your upper torso from side to side.

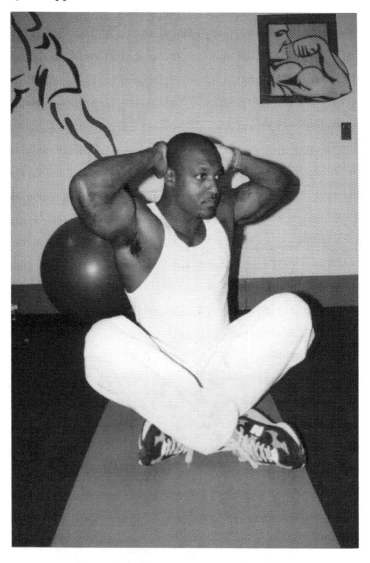

Targets: Abdominal muscles, obliques, and lower back

Stretch 3

Back stretch

While lying on your back, bring both knees toward your chest. Place your hands over your knees and squeeze knees even closer to your chest with light pressure.

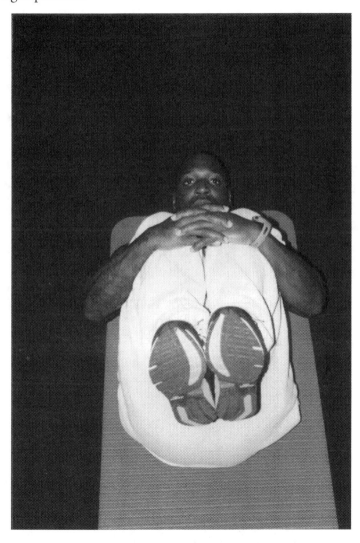

Targets: Back extensor muscles

Stretch 4

Prone stretch, torso

Lie completely on your stomach with your hands flat in front of you like in the push-up position. Extend your arms until your upper torso is completely off the deck while at the same time keeping your hips planted on the floor.

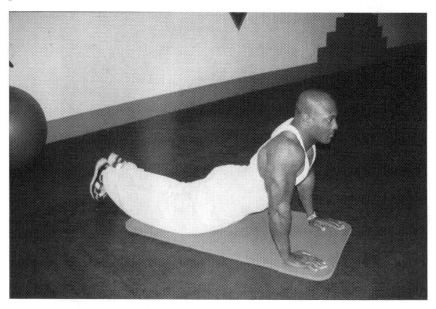

Target: Abdominal muscle

Stretch 5

Adductor stretches

Start in the standing position with your feet spread far apart and toes pointed outward—not too much, but slightly. Shift your body weight to one side while bending the knee of the side you're leaning toward. To avoid stress on knees and joints don't bend the knee of the bent leg further than the alignment over your toe.

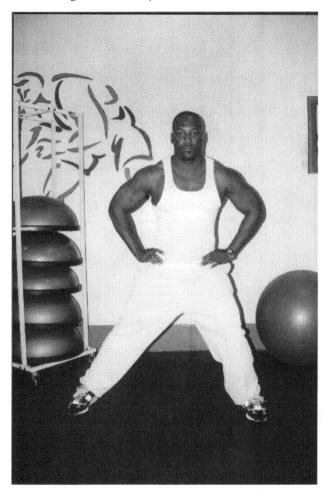

Targets: Hip and leg adductors

Stretch 6

Sitting hamstring stretch

Start in the sitting position with your legs together and straight but with a very slight bend at the knees. Place your hand at your sides while keeping a bend in your upper body; slide your hands forward until you feel the tension build up behind your thighs.

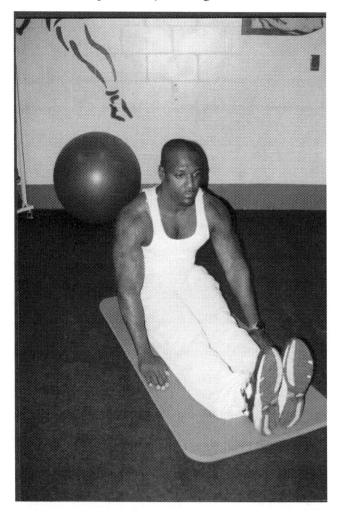

Target: Hamstrings

Chapter 3
The Core/Abs

Let's face it—there's nothing like a flat stomach layered with hard abs! So let's get straight to it! Along with eating properly, doing an abs circuit the correct way is the only way to get the chiseled abs you desire.

It is also good to know that the stronger your core is the stronger your performance will be in all aspects of your workout. If the core is weak, your extremities will not function properly. This may cause muscle imbalances in the kinetic chain.

Many back problems are a direct effect of a weak core. Training that relates to everyday activities and focuses on core stability will improve and enhance your life in every way. To greatly improve your core not only do you have to work at it frequently in the proper manner, but it would be wise to implement medicine balls and free weights into your already existing workout routine as well as dynamic movements; challenge the center of gravity. Doing this will increase the stress in the desired area for greater results.

The end result will be a stronger core! Getting great abs takes a series of different routines that make up a circuit, targeting all the abdominal regions for maximum success.

I guess that puts an end to the old notion that you can do the same routine, such as sit-ups or crunches, day after day—doing these same routines in such great quantity that it's impossible (you think) *not* to get the abs you want. To be honest, that's just not going to happen; no one routine in a repetitive workout will do it. It takes discipline and knowledge of the entire core family.

The good thing about an amazing six-pack is that you're already got it; we just need to get it more defined. The first step is to remember to stay consistent with a healthy diet as I talked about in chapter one; this will help burn away that unwanted fat so you and everyone else can see how all your hard work and efforts have paid off.

Now that we're established the importance of your abdominal area, let me give you a crash course on the major areas of the core region.

Major areas of the core region

Rectus abdominis: This is the muscle that helps in all upper-body movement, such as when you're doing crunches. It's also usually the first part you see when you begin to lose weight in the abdominal area. The rectus abdominis is a thin layer of muscle that's layered over the entire front of your stomach.

External obliques: These are those little knots that you see on the side of your rib cage that extend diagonally down the side of your waist. It's safe to say that the majority of all rotating torso movements, such as those used in golf or any other sport, that require this type of movement rely mainly on the external oblique.

Transverse Abdominis: Commonly referred to as the girdle because of the way it wraps around the midsection, this muscle gives support and stability to the entire midsection.

Now that we've got that out of the way, let's get back to the how and when to work your abdominal area.

Working the abdominal area

First of all, most people trying to get abs are so impatient that they work on their abs every day, and that's not the way to do it. The abs need rest just like every other muscle in your body. They grow when they're at rest, not when you're actually doing the exercises. Work your abs no more than three times a week so you can allow them to grow strong and healthy.

The abs circuit

Now that you've had your crash course in all five regions we move to my second point. When working your abs it is important to work all areas, and the best way to do this is by doing an abs circuit. Choose one routine for each region to make sure you're hitting all areas. With this book you'll have several different exercises to pick from, so mix it up after each workout. You'll see better results by doing this because your abs won't get used to doing the same thing, and change stimulates growth.

When you first start doing the abs circuit do one of each routine one set after the other. As you get better, usually by the second or third week, do two or three of each routine in the same circuit.

Another key to achieving a rock-hard core is to go slow. When you do all your exercises, the slower you do each rep the greater the intensity, and the higher the intensity the stronger the stomach. Doing the reps fast just to get them over with does nothing for you, because all you're doing then is letting the momentum of the motion do all the work and not the actual muscles. Each rep should last at least four to five seconds.

I've set the routines up by the level of difficulty. To do an abs circuit, pick one routine for each region. Pick which routine best fits you, and work them in the order below.

–**Upper Abs**
–**Lower Abs**
–**Obliques**
–**Transverse Abdominis**
–**Lower Back**

Brian Bebley

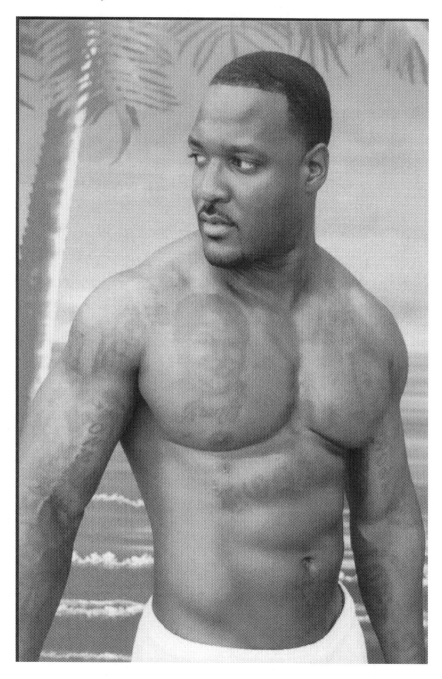

Upper Abs

Lie on your back with your knees up; make sure your knees are close together. Crunch up slowly, bringing your shoulders up off the ground.

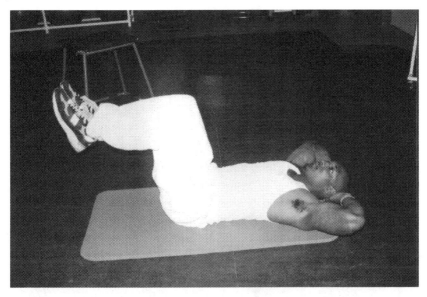

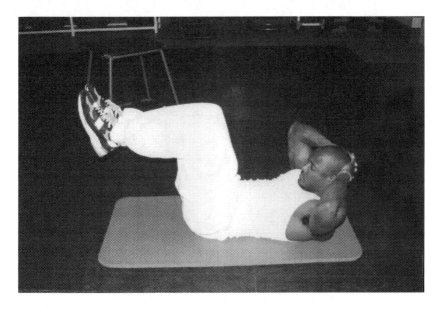

Crunch: Beginner; twelve to fifteen repetitions

Upper Abs

Lie on the floor and cross your legs; raise your feet slightly off the ground. Crunch upward until the outside of your elbows touches your knees, pause, and then repeat the process, never letting your feet touch the ground throughout the entire set.

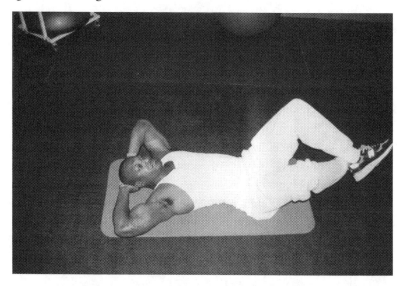

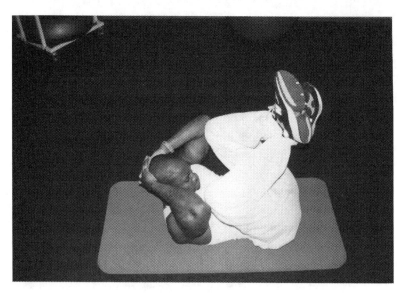

Cross leg crunch: Intermediate; twelve to fifteen repetitions

Upper Abs

Lie on your back with your legs raised straight in the air directly over your hips. Bring your arms straight up and reach toward your toes. The goal is to touch your toes with your fingertips. Use your upper abs to push your body upward. Go slow and repeat process.

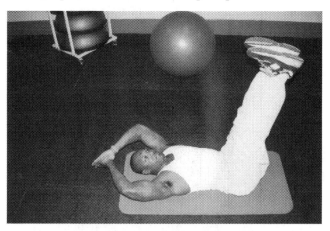

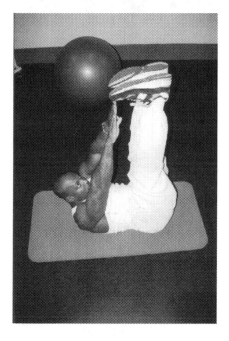

Toe touches: Intermediate; twelve to fifteen repetitions

Upper Abs

Lie on your back with your legs raised straight in the air directly over your hips. Step 1: hold a medicine ball directly over your chest. Step 2: crunch up while pushing the ball toward your toes.

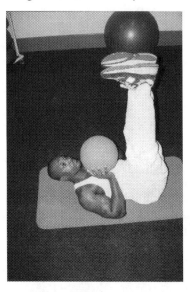

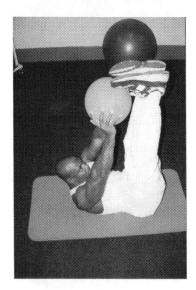

Toe touches with medicine ball: Advanced; twelve to fifteen repetitions

Upper Abs

Lie on your back with your feet planted firmly on the floor. Step 1: hold a medicine ball directly on your chest. Step 2: raise your upper body as high as possible by crunching upward. Steps 3: extend your arms outward with ball, keeping arms straight. Hold for two seconds and repeat routine.

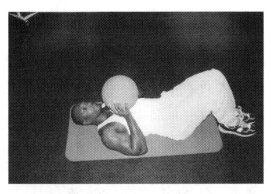

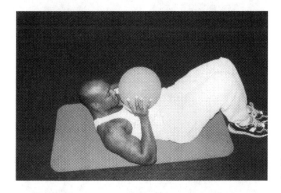

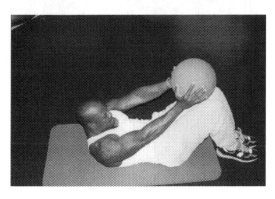

Lower Abs

Lie on your back with your legs and feet completely straight and your arms at your sides for support. Use your lower abdominal to raise your legs up off the floor while keeping them straight. Lower your legs slowly, but don't let your feet touch the ground. Repeat cycle.

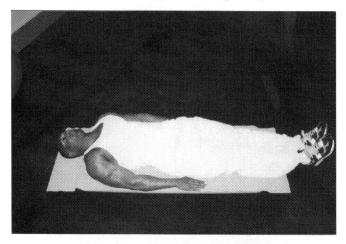

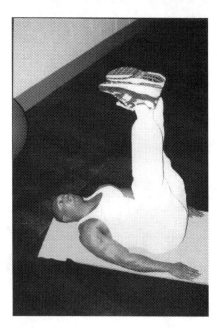

Leg raise: Beginner; twelve to fifteen repetitions

Lower Abs

Sit on the edge of a bench or any stable platform. Place your hands in front of your butt, lean back, and slowly extend your legs in a downward motion, keeping your feet at least five inches off the ground. Slowly bring your knees back up, and in a crunching motion bring your upper body to meet your knees.

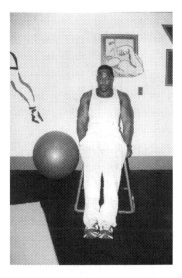

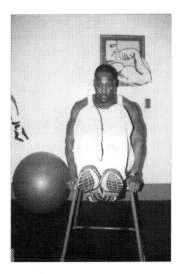

Hanging knee tucks: Intermediate; twelve to fifteen repetitions

Lower Abs

Get a firm grip on the pull-up bar. To prevent shoulder injury, *do not* hang entirely on joints. Bring your knees toward your chest, curling your pelvis upward. Lower your legs slowly so you control your core enough not to swing while hanging on the bar; repeat motion.

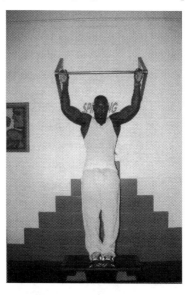

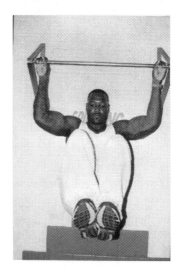

Hanging knee tucks: Intermediate; twelve to fifteen repetitions

Lower Abs

Get a firm grip on the pull-up bar. To prevent shoulder injury, *do not* hang entirely on joints. Bring one knee up at a time, rotating them in a pausing up-and-down motion. Remember to go slowly to control the motion of your torso.

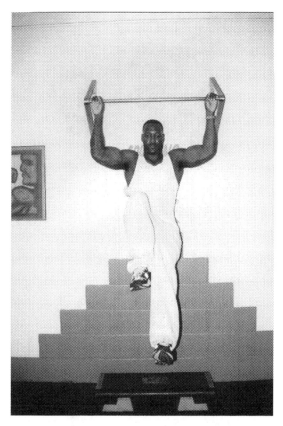

Hanging bicycle: Intermediate; eight repetition on each leg

Lower Abs

Lie down on the floor with a medicine ball held tightly between your calf muscles. Slowly bring your legs straight up right above your hips; pause for one second before lowering legs again. Do not let your feet touch the ground after the first rep.

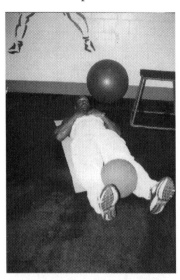

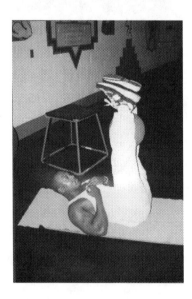

Medicine ball leg raise: Advanced; twelve to fifteen repetitions

Obliques

Lie on your back with your knees up; place one leg over the other with your ankle resting at the top of your thigh. Place your hands behind your head and slowly bring your opposite elbow to meet the top of your knee on the resting leg. Hold for one second at the top and then slowly go back to the starting position.

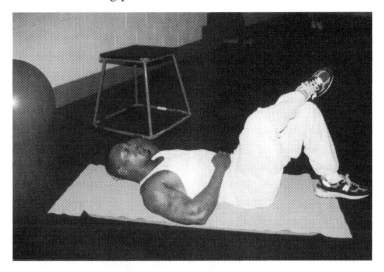

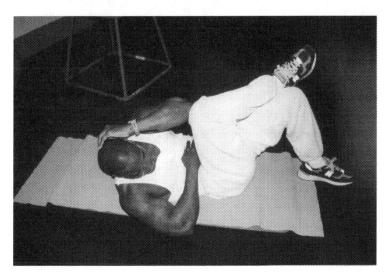

Oblique sit-ups: Beginner; ten repetitions on each side

Obliques

While in the standing position with your feet shoulder-width apart, hold a medicine ball firmly in your hands with your arms extended. Rotate from side to side, going as fast as you can while keeping your back and hips straight and feet planted.

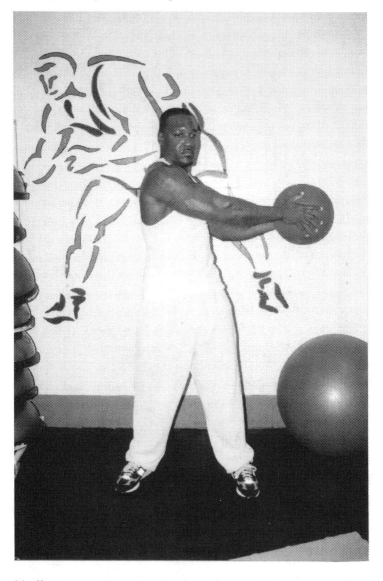

Speed ball: Intermediate; ten repetitions on each side

Obliques

Lie on your side, resting on your hip and forearm with your leg straight. Look forward and keep one hand placed on your hip. Raise your torso and hip off the floor. Pause to feel the contraction on the side of your waist. Slowly lower your hip and torso and then repeat.

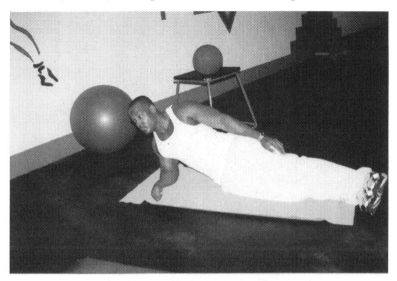

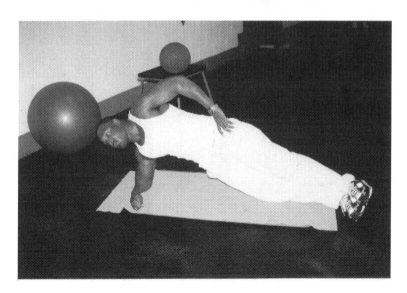

Reverse jackknife: Intermediate; ten repetitions on each side

Obliques

While in the standing position with your feet shoulder-width apart, position yourself three to four feet from the wall. Rotate, while looking back and keeping your feet planted, and release the ball so that it hits the wall. When the ball bounces back catch and quickly rotate to the opposite side and repeat the same motion. The quicker the better!

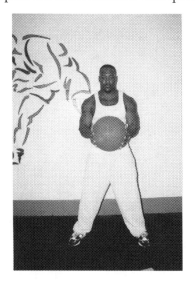

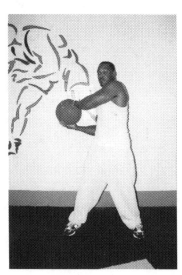

Oblique ball bounce: Advanced; ten repetitions on each side

Transverse Abdominis

Lie on the floor and bring your arms under you until you're supporting your weight on your elbows and toes. Your body should be as straight as possible from the top of your head to your ankles. Hold in this position while pulling your abdominals inward and squeezing as tight as possible. Hold for thirty seconds at a time; as you get stronger try holding this position for sixty seconds at a time.

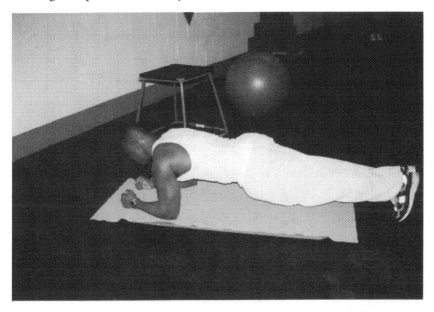

The plank: Beginner

Transverse Abdominis

Sit on the floor with your feet spread shoulder-width apart and your knees bent. Extend your arms out with your palms down, one hand over the other. Your upper body should be in a slightly ninety degree angle to the floor in the starting position. Lower your body toward the floor while tightening your stomach and crunching your upper body until you round your back off. When you're a few inches from the floor return to the starting position while keeping your stomach tight the entire time.

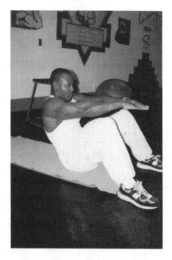

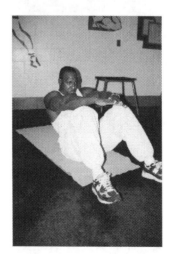

Transverse negative crunch: Intermediate; twelve repetitions

Transverse Abdominis

Start in the push-up position with your hands shoulder-width apart while resting your shin on a Swiss ball. Keep your back completely flat from head to toe. Roll the ball toward your chest, hold in this position for a second, and then return the ball to its starting position.

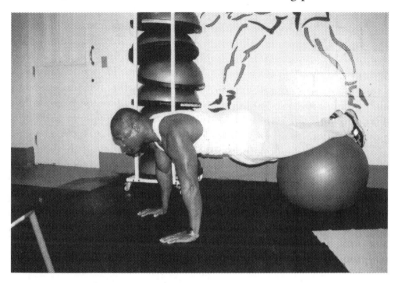

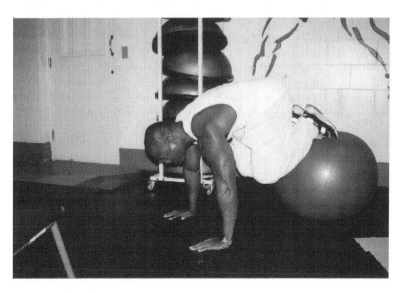

Swiss ball roll: Intermediate; eight to ten repetitions

Transverse Abdominis

Kneel on the floor, using a towel or mat to support your knees. Using the wheel, roll out almost until you're fully extended. Slowly roll back to the starting position.

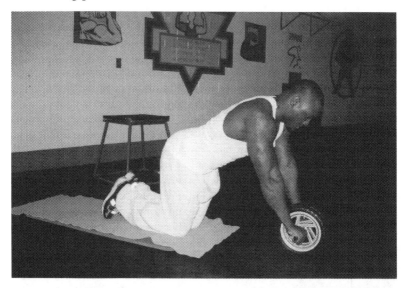

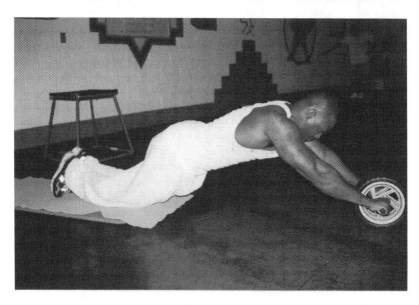

Wheel roll: Advanced; twelve to fifteen repetitions

Lower Back

Lie on your back with your knees bent and your feet flat on the floor. Do a crunch while tightening up your abdominal area. Keeping your shoulders off the floor and your chest high, do a backstroke with one arm at a time, flexing your torso toward the outstretched arm. The higher you can lift your shoulders off the floor the more intense your workout will be.

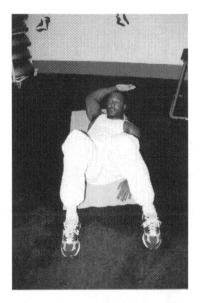

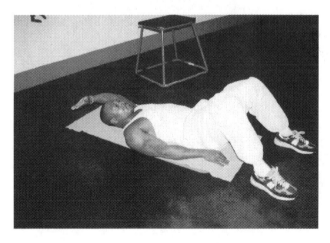

Lower backstrokes: Intermediate to advanced; five to ten repetitions

Lower Back

Lay crouched over a Swiss ball with your legs straight, shoulder-width apart, and your toes braced on the floor. Tuck your elbows in and place your hands on the sides of your head. Slowly raise your torso off the ball, extending your arms out at the same time. Once your body is straight from your fingertips to your ankles, hold in this position and then slowly pull back to the starting position.

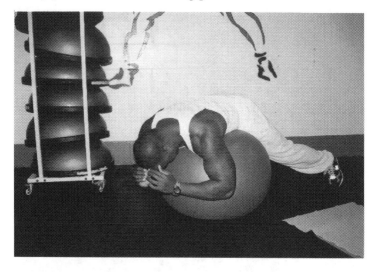

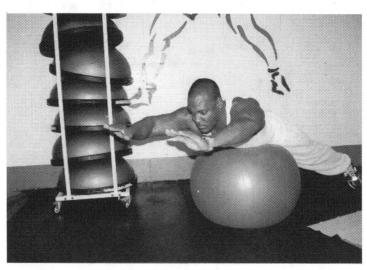

Superman back extension: Intermediate; twelve to fifteen repetitions

Four gladiator abs routine

Do you want to be able to build your abdominis to be as hard as steel, tougher than granite, as firm as oak?

I'm assuming you're saying yes; then I have the right plan for you. Along with the Abs routine previously shown, in these next pages I'll demonstrate four gladiator routines that will intensely work several areas of your midsection simultaneously.

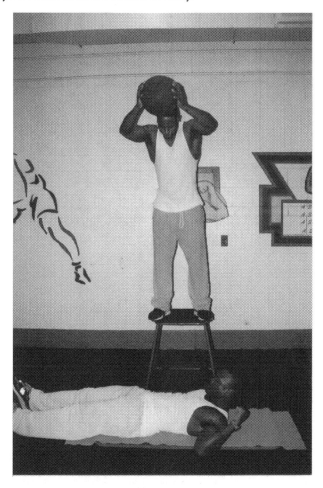

though I can withstand the impact of this 161 lb medicine ball from over eight feet in the air without even wincing, I don't recommend that you try this at home; this is just a demonstration to show you just how solid your core *will* be!

Multi-Abs Routine
Upper and Lower Crunch

Lie on the floor with your feet and upper body completely straight. Place your hands on the sides of your head. Simultaneously lift your legs and torso until they meet in the center, pause for two to three seconds, and then slowly lower your legs and torso back into the starting position. Note: for added intensity never let your feet touch the ground after your first rep.

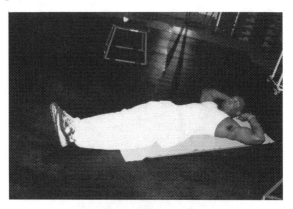

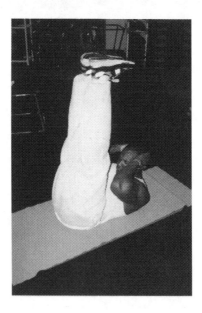

Target: Lower and upper abs; ten to fifteen repetitions

Multi-Abs Routine
Cross Leg Crunch

Lie on the floor with your hands behind your head. Place one leg in the figure-four pattern over the other leg. Make sure your ankle is positioned just below the kneecap of the straight leg. Once you have proper form, simultaneously bring your straightened leg to a tucked position while keeping your crossed leg in place. Pause for two to three seconds and then repeat, alternating between sets with each leg.

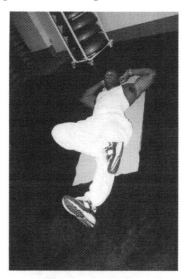

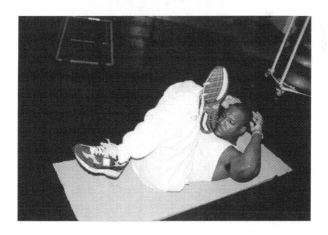

Target: Lower and upper abs; ten to fifteen repetitions

Multi-Abs Routine
Bicycle Rotating Crunch

Lie on your back with your hands behind your head and your legs completely straight. In one motion bring your right leg up and bring your left elbow to meet your knee. Note: pay attention to the form illustrated in the picture. Once you've paused for a brief moment in this position slowly return to the starting position and then rotate up again, this time using your right elbow to meet your left knee.

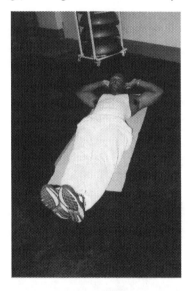

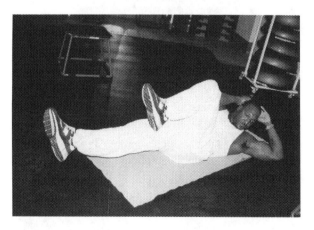

Target: Obliques, upper and lower abs; ten to sixteen repetitions

Multi-Abs Routine
Hanging Knee Twist

Get a firm grip on the pull-up bar, hang down just enough not to cause a shoulder injury, and maintain your balance and form while keeping legs straight. Slowly bring one knee up while at the same time twisting toward the opposite side, pause, and then return to the starting position before raising the other knee.

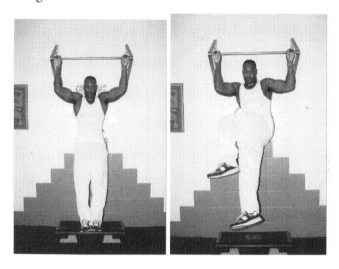

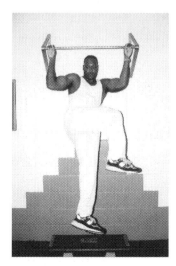

Target: Obliques, transverse and lower abs; four to eight repetitions

Chapter 4
Circuit Training

Whether your goal is to maintain lean muscle mass or lose body fat there is no substitute for circuit training. Circuit training allows you to use the most body parts during a workout while burning more calories than you could doing single-section or isolation workouts.

You should never try to isolate muscles when circuit training. Instead you should get as many muscle groups going as possible while maintaining good posture and form. This will allow for a balanced training session.

The main purpose of circuit training besides the obvious one of losing weight is to increase your heart rate while using some form of resistance.

While circuit training, the object is to keep moving so that you maintain your target heart rate. This aspect of circuit training is crucial!

In this book you'll find several examples of non-free-weight exercises to pick from to put together the right or ideal circuit routine that best fits you. Always keep in mind while choosing the circuit routine that's best for you that your circuit training session should involve as many major muscle groups as possible. So pick one routine from each group of demonstration pictures to form a complete circuit.

I have indicated a level of difficulty for each of the routines for the circuit. Beginners will naturally start with the beginning exercises; as you grow stronger and more confident in your ability to perform greater and more difficult exercises you can select routines from the advanced section.

Posture and form is an absolute must! Maintaining them appropriately will prevent all sorts of unnecessary injuries. It is also imperative that all movements are done in a slow and controlled manner; adding a one-second pause while doing all reps will stimulate muscle growth.

A prime mover is a muscle group that is directly responsible for the movement of resistance in a given exercise. Your body has a functional capacity of some 656 individual muscles.

Muscles hardly ever work alone. They can get shorter and pull, but they cannot push, so note that muscles are arranged in opposing groups. One group pulls the body part one way while the other group pulls it back again. As one group pulls, the other group relaxes and is stretched while doing so.

Approximately 60 percent of the total number of cells in the body are muscle tissue cells.

Now back to the point of circuit training. The more muscle you have the more fat your body is able to burn. Now that we know that over half of our body cells are made up of muscle it is clear that it is reasonable to get as many of these muscles involved as possible in all circuit training sessions.

With your newfound knowledge of muscles and circuit training I am sure you will apply this to your workout for maximum results. The fact that you're even reading this book is a testimony to your desire to excel in your goal to lose weight or get ripped!

I have no doubt in my mind and am fully confident that if you follow this basic format you will reach your goal!

The pectorals major and minor, triceps, and deltoids are worked during most pushing and pressing exercises. The primary muscle group that is stressed doing push-ups is the pectorals.

Standard Push-ups

Place your hands on the floor shoulder-width apart for the starting position; keep the entire body in line and straight. Now press your body to the full extension of your arms while keeping your body straight, paying close attention to the lower back to avoid injury. Slowly lower your body and then repeat.

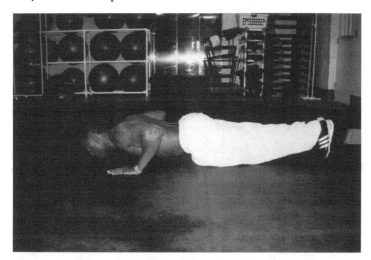

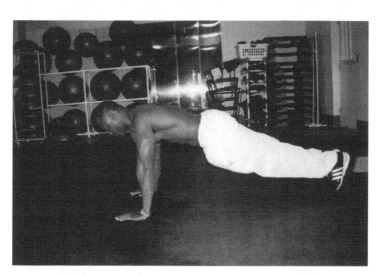

Beginner: Ten to twenty repetitions
Targets: Pectorals and triceps

Diamond Push-up

Start in the standard push-up position with both your hands together in the diamond shape directly under your chest, thumbs touching and pointer fingers touching. Breathe out deeply while fully extending your body upward. Slowly lower your body to the starting position and then repeat.

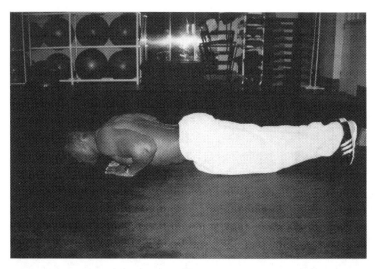

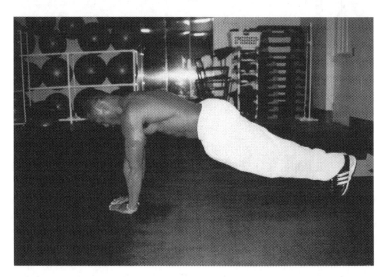

Beginner/Intermediate: *to twelve repetitions
Targets: Pectorals and triceps

Upper Elevated Push-up

Place your hands on a sturdy platform in the standard push-up position while keeping your body straight. Breathe out and fully extend your arms until your body is straight. Slowly lower your body until your chest touches the platform and then repeat.

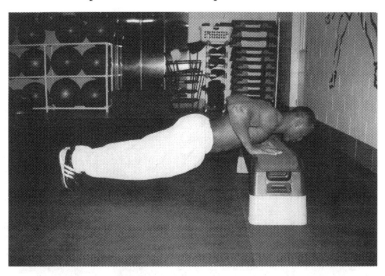

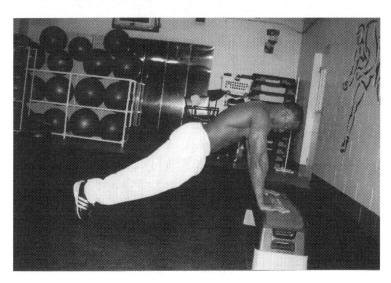

Intermediate: Ten to fifteen repetitions
Targets: Pectorals and triceps

Lower Elevated Push-ups

Start in the standard push-up position, but with your feet elevated on a step, chair, or bench. Fully extend your arms until your body is elevated completely off the ground. Note: it is critical to keep your back straight in this position to avoid injury. Lower your body slowly and then repeat.

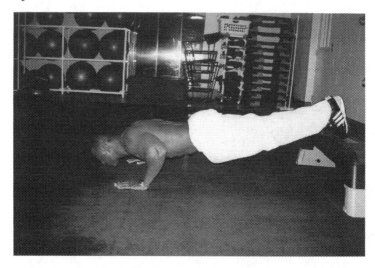

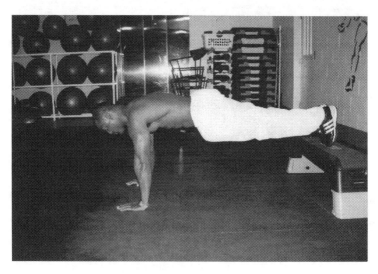

Intermediate/Advanced: Eight to twelve repetitions
Targets: Pectoral and triceps

Medicine Ball Push-ups

Start out by placing two evenly weighted medicine balls shoulder-width apart. Place your hands directly on top of the balls while lowering yourself slowly in the center of the balls. Slowly extend your arms while keeping your body straight. Tighten your midsection to get the full effect. Slowly lower your back down and then repeat.

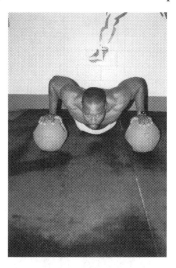

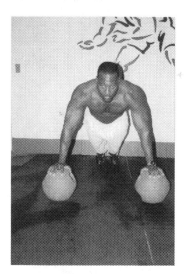

Advanced: Eight to ten repetitions
Targets: Pectorals, triceps, and core

Lateral Raise

Hold dumbbells or medicine balls with your hand grips at each side and elbows slightly bent toward the center of your body. Raise your arms slowly without using momentum until your arms are parallel to the floor. Contract your shoulders muscles, and then lower your arms back down to your sides.

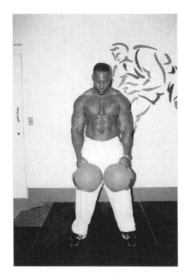

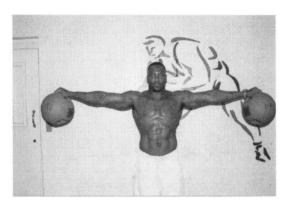

Eight to ten repetitions
Target: Triceps
The latissimus dorsi, teres majors and minor, rhomboids, and biceps are the major groups affected or worked during pulling and rowing movements.

Standard Pull-ups

Start by getting a firm grip on the pull-up bar, placing your hands a little wider than shoulder-width. Pull your body upward without jerking your body and using the momentum to propel you upward; instead concentrate on using your back and arms. Slowly lower your body back down and then repeat.

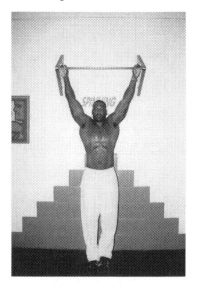

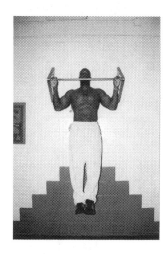

Beginner: Five to ten repetitions
Targets: Biceps and latissimus dorsi

Roman Chair Pull-ups

Place your hands shoulder-width apart and get a firm grip on the pull-up bar. Note: to avoid injury do not hang completely on your shoulders. Bring your knees up into a chair position. Pull your body upward while keeping your core tight, squeeze the muscles in your back when you get to the top of the rep, slowly lower your body, and then repeat while keeping your legs in the seated position.

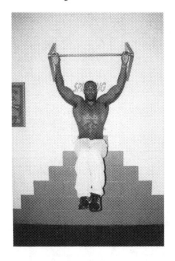

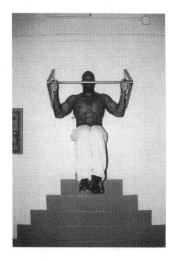

Intermediate: Five to ten repetitions
Target: Biceps, latissimus dorsi, and core

Bicep Curl Pull-ups

Place your hands in an underhand position about six inches apart for added effect; slowly bring your chin up and over the pull-up bar. Slowly lower your body and then repeat.

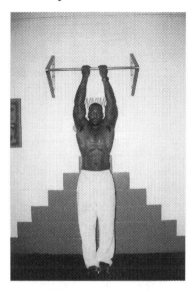

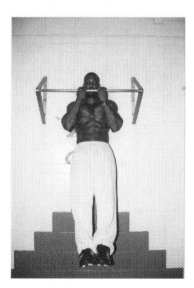

Intermediate: Five to ten repetitions
Targets: Biceps and latissimus dorsi

Elevated Leg Pull-ups

Place your hands a little wider than shoulder width and get a firm grip on the pull-up bar. Slowly raise your legs until they are parallel to the floor, keeping your ankles together and legs straight. Do a pull-up while holding in this position. *Note:* keep your entire midsection tight through each rep. Slowly lower your body while keeping your legs straight and then repeat.

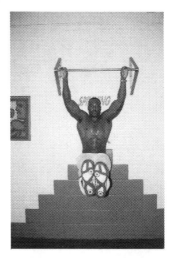

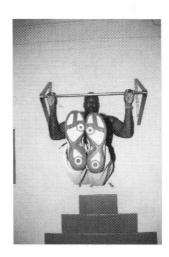

Advanced: Five to ten repetitions
Targets: Biceps, latissimus dorsi, and core

The Cranking Back

Using a dumbbell or medicine ball with handgrips, hold firmly in one hand and place your opposite hand and knee on a fitness step or bench. Keeping your back straight and parallel to the floor, bring the weight up toward your chest, keeping it on the side of your body as you bring it up, pausing for a second and contracting your back muscles. Lower the weight slowly and then repeat in a controlled motion.

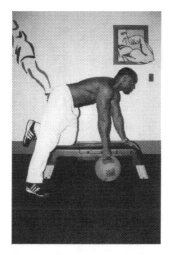

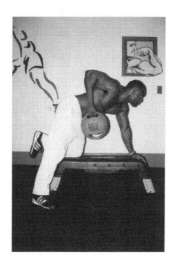

Targets: Trapezius (traps), latissimus dorsi, deltoids
Eight to ten repetitions on each side

Standard Squat

Place your hands on your hips while standing upright with your feet shoulder-width apart. Lower your body until your upper thighs are parallel to the floor. Keep your back straight while keeping your lower back arched in throughout the entire motion.

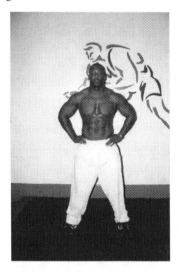

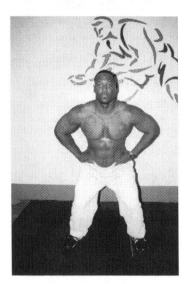

Beginner: Ten to twenty repetitions
Target: Quadriceps

Concentrated Squats

Place your feet side by side, leaving little or no space at all between them; keep your knees together. For added resistance use dumbbells or a medicine ball with handgrips to maximize stress on your prime movers (quads). While keeping your hands at your side lower your body while keeping your back straight and lower back arched in a natural way. Pause when you've reached the point when you can't go down any further; then slowly stand up to the starting position.

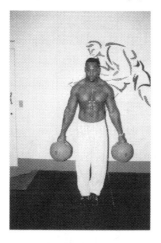

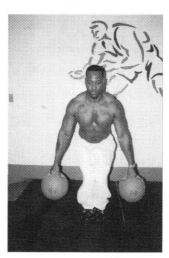

Intermediate/Advanced: Ten to twenty repetitions
Target: Quadriceps

Leg Lunges with Medicine Ball

Stand straight up with your feet about a foot apart, using dumbbells or medicine balls with handgrips. Keep your arms straight down by your sides. Step forward until the quad of your outstretched leg is parallel to the floor, pause for one second, and then return to starting position before switching legs.

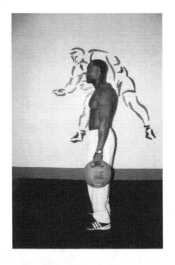

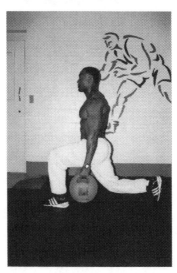

Intermediate: Ten to twenty repetitions
Targets: Quadriceps, hamstrings, and glutes

Concentrated Lunges with Feet Elevated/Lateral Raise

Stand directly in front of an aerobic step and bring one leg back until your toe is resting on top of the step. Lower your body while simultaneously raising the medicine ball until your arms are parallel to the ground, pause, and then slowly stand to the starting position while lowering the medicine ball gradually as you stand up.

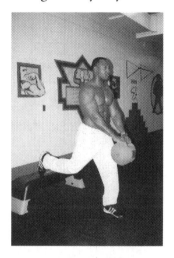

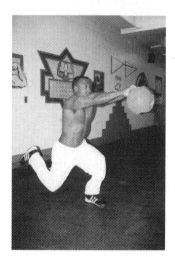

Advanced: Eight to twelve repetition on each leg
Target: Quadriceps, hamstrings, glutes, and deltoids

W-A-T-E-R!!!!!

Where do I start? Water is the most vital component in synovial fluid, which is a joint lubricant, and cerebrospinal fluid in the nervous system.

Sixty percent of your body weight is water; it also helps with circulation, digestion, the movement of vital nutrients for your body, and the removal of wastes.

Despite what has been previously said from other sources of information, cold water is the best. The colder the water the better. Cold water is absorbed in the small intestine faster, making it better for you before, during, and after your workouts.

The best way to accurately fulfill your water needs after working out is to weigh yourself before you work out and then drink sixteen ounces of water per pound of weight lost, at a rate of eight ounces every twenty minutes.

How to put together your abs circuit and total body circuit routine

Example of a total body workout

A circuit training routine can be done at least three to four times a week. Also, an abs circuit incorporated into your circuit is an effective way to lose weight, build muscle, and chisel your core out!

Abs circuit	Reps	Sets
Upper abs	12–15	1
Lower abs	12–15	1
Obliques	10 on each side	1
Transverse Abs	12–15	1
Lower back	12–15	1

Rest for two minutes before starting total body circuit

Total body circuit	Reps	Sets
	5–10	3–5 of each routine you've selected

Repeat this cycle throughout the week while taking the day off mentioned earlier.

Note: I've chosen light cardiovascular exercise for you twice a week. This will also help you to reach your goal of losing weight and getting ripped. Also remember to change routines for each circuit every day; this will stimulate muscle growth. As you get stronger you can go from doing one set of each routine to two or three sets per abs and a total body circuit routine.

Circuit Training: The best way to do a circuit training routine is several sets of a pushing movement, a pulling movement, and a lower body movement.
Allow one to three minutes between sets for lactic acid removal.

Lactic Acid: Accumulates in muscle fiber during intense workout, blocking complete contractions; also known as the pump. It can be converted back into energy by the liver.

Example of a workout program

Monday: Abs circuit and total body circuit

Tuesday: Light cardio such as walking, swimming, or slow jogging for no longer than thirty-five minutes

Wednesday: Abs circuit and total body circuit

Thursday: Light cardio, the same as Tuesday, for at least thirty minutes

Friday: Abs circuit and total body circuit

Saturday: Light cardio

Sunday: (Off)

Remember that you can change this schedule around, but keep in mind that you need at least two cardio days and at least one day for total rest. Also give yourself a day between each total body workout for maximum progress.

Most commonly used foods for diet preparation

Proteins, carbohydrates, and fats appear on this chart in grams.

Sugars	Serving	Protein	Carb	Fat	Cal
Honey	1T	0.1	17.8	0	64
Sucrose (Table sugar)	1T	0	4	0	16
Fructose (Fruit sugar)	1T	0	4	0	15

Beverages	Serving	Protein	Carb	Fat	Cal
Coffee	6 oz	–	0.54	0.01	3
Soda	12 oz	–	40	–	159
Diet Soda	12 oz	–	0.43	–	1
Vegetable Juice	1 c	2.2	4.7	0.2	41

Condiments	Serving	Protein	Carb	Fat	Cal
Butter	1 T	0.12	0.01	11.5	101
Olive oil	1 T	0	0	14	120
Jelly	1 T	0.1	12.7	0	49
Syrup	2 T	0	25.6	0	100
Ketchup	1 T	0.3	3.8	0.1	16
Mustard	1 T	0.9	0.9	0.9	15
Mayonnaise	1 T	0.2	0.4	11	99
Tartar Sauce	1 T	0.1	0.09	3.1	31
Soy Sauce	1 T	1.56	1.5	0	12

Dairy	Serving	Protein	Carb	Fat	Cal
Ice Cream	1 c	4.8	31.7	14.3	269
Yogurt (plain)	1 c	7.9	10.5	7.4	139
Yogurt (Low-Fat plain)	1 c	11.9	16	3.52	144

Whole Milk	8 oz	8.03	11.37	8.15	150
Skim Milk	8 oz	8.35	11.8	0.44	86
Eggs, Whole	11 g	6.07	0.6	5.58	79
Egg, White	11 g	3.35	0.41	—	16
Cheddar Cheese	1 oz	7.06	0.36	9.4	114
Swiss Cheese	1 oz	8.06	0.96	7.78	107
Mozzarella Cheese	1 oz	5.5	0.63	6.12	80
Cottage Cheese, 2% milk	1 c	31	8.2	4.36	152
Cream Cheese	1 oz	2.14	0.75	9.9	99
Parmesan Cheese	1 T	2	0.19	1.5	23
Sour Cream	1 c	7.27	9.82	48.2	493

Fruits	**Serving**	**Protein**	**Carb**	**Fat**	**Cal**
Bananas	1	1.8	26.7	0.55	105
Grapes	1 c	1.06	28.4	0.92	114
Oranges	1	1.23	15.4	0.16	62
Apples	1	0.27	21	0.49	81
Pears	1	0.65	25	0.66	98
Grapefruit	½	0.75	9.7	0.12	38
Plum	1	0.52	8.59	0.41	36
Cherries	1 c	1.74	24	1.39	104
Strawberries	1 c	0.91	10.4	0.55	45
Blueberries	1 c	0.97	20.5	0.55	82
Apricots	5	1.5	26.3	–	105
Dates	10	1.63	61	0.37	228
Raisin	½ c	3	54.5	–	230
Figs	10	5.7	109	2.18	477
Prunes	10	2.19	52.7	0.43	201
Melon, cantaloupes	½	2.34	22.3	0.97	94
Honeydew	½	1.18	23.6	1.54	92
Watermelon	½	0.99	11.5	0.48	50

Vegetables	Serving	Protein	Carb	Fat	Cal
Potato	11 g	4	32.8	02	210
Carrots	½ c	0.5	5.5	0.1	24
Beets	1 c	2	13.6	0.2	60
Sweet Corn	1 c	4.96	29	1.8	132
Peas	1 c	7.9	21	0.59	118
Yams	1 c	4.8	48.2	0.4	210
Sweet Potato	1	2	32	0.38	136
Green Beans	1 c	2	8	0.01	34
Broccoli	1 c	2.6	4.6	0.3	24
Cauliflower	1 c	1.98	4.9	0.18	24
Mushrooms	1 c	1.5	3	0.3	18
Lettuce, Iceberg	1 c	0.7	2.2	0.12	10
Lettuce, Romaine	1 c	0.9	1.3	0.12	8
Tomato	1	1.1	5	0.26	24
Sweet Pepper	1 c	0.86	5.3	0.46	24

Dried Legumes	Serving	Protein	Carb	Fat	Cal
Butter beans	8 oz	12	30	0	200
Lima beans	1 c	11.6	40	0.54	208
Black-eyed peas	1 c	13.2	29.9	1.3	178
Kidney beans	1 c	14.4	39.6	0.9	218
Lentils	1 c	15.6	38.6	–	212
Navy beans	1 c	14.8	40.3	1.1	224
Pinto beans	1 c	13	40.8	1.4	224
Great Northern beans	1 c	12.8	40.8	1.2	228

Breakfast cereals	Serving	Protein	Carb	Fat	Cal
Cornflakes, Kellogg's	1	1.84	19.5	0.08	88

	Serving	Protein	Carb	Fat	Cal
Shredded wheat, Quaker	2	5	31	1	160
Wheat, puffed	1 c	1.8	9.5	0.1	44
Mueslix, Kellogg	½ c	3	31	2	130
Mueslix, five grain	½ c	4	32	1	140
All-Bran, Kellogg	1/3 c	4	22	1.1	114
Bran flakes, 40% post	1 c	5.3	37.3	0.8	152
Oatmeal, total	1/3 c	4	19	2	100
Rice, puffed	1 c	0.9	12.6	0.1	56

Grain; cereal products	Serving	Protein	Carb	Fat	Cal
White rice, enriched	½ c	6.55	78.5	0.75	354
White rice, minute	½ c–ckd	2	20	0	90
Whole wheat bread	1 sl	2.4	11	0.7	56
Honey wheat bran, Grants	1 sl	3	13	1	70
White Bread, enriched	1 sl	2	11.6	0.79	62
Brown rice	½ c	7.4	76	1.8	352
White Spaghetti; dry	2 oz	7	42	1	210
Whole wheat spaghetti	4 oz	20	78	1	400

Bagels/Muffins	Serving	Protein	Carb	Fat	Cal
Bagel, plain	1	11	56	2.57	296
English muffin, enriched	1	7	4	1	130

Nuts	Serving	Protein	Carb	Fat	Cal
Peanuts	1 c	37.7	29.7	70.1	838
Sunflower seeds	½ c	17.4	14.4	34.3	406
Almonds	1 c	26.4	27.7	77	849
Brazil nuts	1 c	20	15.3	93.7	916

Cashew, nuts	1 c	24.1	41	64	78.5

Beef	Serving	Protein	Carb	Fat	Cal
Hamburger	8 oz	40.6	–	48.1	608
Steak, sirloin	7 oz	31.1	–	49	576
Steak, T-Bone	7 oz	25.8	–	73.5	698
Steak, porterhouse	8 oz	30.5	–	74	802
Roast beef	8 oz	33.5	–	43.7	580

Luncheon meat/ Sausage	Serving	Protein	Carb	Fat	Cal
Ham	4 oz	19.9	3.5	12	207
Bologna, beef	1 oz	3.31	0.55	8.04	89
Bologna, pork	1 oz	4.34	0.21	5.63	70
Salami, hard	1/16" sl	2.29	0.26	3.44	42
Pepperoni	1 sl	1.15	0.16	2.42	27
Sausages, Polish	1 oz	4	0.46	8.14	92
Bacon	4 oz	9.75	0.11	65.3	631
Pork chop	1	20	–	29.2	345

Poultry	Serving	Protein	Carb	Fat	Cal
Chicken, white	4 oz	23.5	–	3.2	216
Chicken, white, skinned	4 oz	20.4	–	.36	100
Chicken, dark	4 oz	26.7	–	7.33	379
Chicken, dark, skinned	4 oz	21.9	–	1.18	136
Turkey, white	4 oz	39.0	–	3.3	286
Turkey, dark	4 oz	28.7	–	3.33	243

Seafood	Serving	Protein	Carb	Fat	Cal
Shrimp	8 oz	41	3.4	1.8	207

Lobster	8 oz	38.35	1.15	4.3	207
Cod	8 oz	39.9	–	1.66	177
Halibut	8 oz	47	–	2.5	227
Salmon	8 oz	51	–	30.4	492
Trout	8 oz	48.75	–	25.85	443
Tuna, water pk	½ can	20	–	1.6	99